Yoga and Superfoods

The Power Duo to Optimal Health

Table of Contents

Chapter 1. Introduction

Unleash the power of the ultimate symbiosis between mind, body, and nutrition! In our exclusive special report, "Yoga and Superfoods: The Power Duo to Optimal Health", we unfurl the profound synergy of yoga and superfoods. Delight in learning not only how this potent pair promotes renewed energy, radiant health, and unparalleled longevity, but also how effortlessly you can incorporate them into your daily life. It's not all technical and dull, but a vibrant journey that explores sustenance from the garden and wisdom from the ancients, both blended into an enchanting elixir of life. Continue reading to witness an astonishing transformation that brings together holistic well-being and compelling nutrition. Trust us, this vibrant, easily digestible report is worth its weight in goji berries and kale! Your journey to peak wellness starts here! Invest in our special report and start reshaping your life today!

Chapter 2. Unravelling the Mystique: Yoga and Superfoods Explained

In unraveling the complex bond that exists between yoga and superfoods, we must first delve into the unique components that file each onto the pedestal of health.

2.1. Understanding Yoga

Hailing from ancient India, yoga is a rich amalgamation of physical, mental, and spiritual practices. Initially used as a means to attain spiritual enlightenment, yoga has now enveloped the global holistic health sphere. Its focus on physical postures, meditation, and ethical principles bring a host of rejuvenating benefits, from improved flexibility to a focused mind and nourished spirit.

The central premise of yoga lies in harmonizing these three facets of our being—the physical, mental, and spiritual—portraying a holistic image of health. This unity brings about an equilibrium that bestows a restorative balance in all life areas, inviting tranquility and strength alike.

2.2. Taking a Glimpse at Superfoods

Meanwhile, in the realm of nutrition, superfoods are causing an exciting commotion. While there's no scientific definition, the term generally refers to nutrient-rich foods classified as particularly beneficial for health and wellness.

What exactly do superfoods offer? Simply put, they're a natural powerhouse. Enriched with vitamins, minerals, antioxidants, fiber, and other valuable nutrients, they bolster our body's immunity, combat diseases, spur cognitive function, boost energy levels, and initiate the replenishing process from within.

Pulling from a list that includes foods like goji berries, salmon, kale, and cacao, the range of advantages they offer is remarkable. Be it heart health, weight management, skin vitality, or improved digestion, these nutritional giants have an evident impact.

2.3. The Inextricable Link: Yoga and Superfoods

With mutual standpoints on holistic wellness, it is plain to see why yoga and superfoods form such a symbiotic relationship. Like a glowing sun complements the nurturing soil, they enhance each other—yoga nurturing the mind and body, and superfoods nourishing the body and soul.

The profound synergy lies in the way each calls for a long-term commitment, a sustained lifestyle change. Retaining the beneficial attributes of both requires a steady incorporation into one's daily routine, rather than transient flirtation.

Additionally, both yoga and superfoods cater to individual needs - personalized nutrition meets personalized well-being.

2.4. Amplifying Health Benefits with Yoga and Superfoods

When you blend yoga with superfoods, you are architecting a regime that magnifies each's rewards. Yoga's physical aspect promotes better digestion and absorption of nutrients from superfoods. On the other hand, essential antioxidants, vitamins, and minerals from superfoods refuel the body, bettering the yoga outcomes.

The meditative aspects of yoga guide the mind towards mindful eating, promoting better choices, while the energy from superfoods facilitates improved wellness and yogic endurance.

2.5. Adapting Yoga and Superfoods to Daily Life

You don't need to turn your life upside down to incorporate yoga and superfoods. Start with basic yoga stretches in the morning, even a few minutes can make a marked difference. Pair this with superfood-infused meals throughout the day. By gradually increasing the yoga duration, and weaving in more superfoods into meals, you hit two targets with one effort—a fortified body and an invigorated mind.

It takes time and commitment, but as you cultivate this lifestyle, the transformation in your energy, health, and longevity becomes significantly apparent.

2.6. Choosing the Right Yoga and Superfood Pairing

Not all yoga practices or superfoods have the same effects. Hence, personal understanding becomes crucial in choosing a path that aligns with your life goals and needs.

Explore various yoga forms - such as Hatha, Ashtanga, or Kundalini - and pairing these with different superfoods like chia seeds, goji berries, or kale. Experiment and observe how each combination makes you feel, then tweak accordingly.

The journey to optimal health is never a set path—it's one of exploration and adjustment, and the fusion of yoga and superfoods is no exception.

In the end, unraveling the mystique surrounding yoga and superfoods means grasping their inherent essence as tools for overall health promotion. They are only baffling until you make the first move towards the change. Once the unraveling starts, there is no stopping in the transformative journey ahead. With yoga and superfoods by your side, your health goals cease to be daunting—they become achievable aspirations.

Chapter 3. Harmony Anew: Understanding the Connection

In the harmonious pairing of Yoga and Superfoods, an eloquent language of wellness is woven. This beautiful convergence of disciplined movement and nourishing sustenance provides a robust platform for optimal human health. Delving deeper, we can better appreciate the intricate ties that bind these elements together in a seamless dance of rejuvenation.

3.1. The Essence of Yoga

Yoga, an ancient practice that originates from India, is much more than a series of physical exercises. It's a holistic discipline that unifies the body, mind, and spirit. At its core, Yoga encourages inner peace, emotional stability, mental clarity, and physical strength and flexibility. It does this by focusing on posture (asana), meditation (dhyana), breath control (pranayama), ethical living, and self-realization.

Pranayama, for instance, teaches controlled breathing, which aids in decreasing anxiety, improving cardiovascular health, and enhancing overall energy and mood. Asana helps to fortify muscles, enhance flexibility and posture, contribute to bone health, improve balance, and offer therapeutic benefits for conditions such as arthritis, back pain, and fibromyalgia. Meanwhile, Dhyana enriches mental clarity, fosters emotional stability, reduces stress, increases self-awareness, and inspires a profound sense of harmony within oneself.

A regular yoga practice, thus, can lead to an incredible transformation in physical strength, mental resilience, and oh-so-crucial emotional well-being.

3.2. Confluence with Superfoods

As remarkable as yoga is on its own, combining it with a diet that includes a variety of Superfoods catapults the benefits to a whole new level. Superfoods, a term that's gained popularity in recent years, refers to nutrient-dense foods that are packed with antioxidants, vitamins, and minerals—vital components for maintaining and enhancing human health.

Superfoods range from fresh fruits like blueberries, pomegranates, and avocados to vegetables, grains, and seeds like Kale, Quinoa, and Chia seeds. They also include certain types of fish like salmon and mackerel, nuts like walnuts and almonds, and even dark chocolate.

These power-packed foods provide the body with a full spectrum of essential nutrients, contributing toward fortifying the immune system, boosting energy levels, reducing inflammation, improving brain function, and aiding digestion—just to name a few. Even more, these nutrient-rich champions assist in the battle against a multitude of diseases, such as cancer, heart disease, diabetes, and osteoporosis.

Rather intriguingly, these Superfoods not only enrich our physical health but, in pairing with Yoga, also bolster our mental and spiritual well-being. Foods rich in Vitamin B6, Omega-3 fatty acids, and Tryptophan—such as bananas, salmon, and turkey—support serotonin production, a neurotransmitter that aids in mood regulation and plays a crucial role in managing anxiety and depression. Subsequently, a diet laden with Superfoods can optimize yoga-induced tranquility, resulting in a truly harmonious mind-body connection.

3.3. Synergising Yoga and Superfoods in Everyday Life

In actualizing the synergy between yoga and Superfoods, it becomes crucial to establish a routine accommodating both elements. Begin with a simple, feasible yoga routine and steadily incorporate the different aspects of pranayama, asana, and dhyana. Yoga doesn't demand extraordinary flexibility or Herculean strength; it only requires your willingness, commitment, and consistency.

On the nutrition front, shift towards including more Superfoods in your diet. A handful of almonds for a snack, a glass of blueberry smoothie for breakfast, or a side of steamed kale with your dinner all constitute simple yet powerful ways to start. The journey towards optimal health isn't about revamping your life overnight, but about taking small, sustainable steps daily.

3.4. In Conclusion

Engulfed in the hustle and bustle of modern life, it can be easy to undermine the importance of holistic well-being. Yet this delicate balance between mind, body, and nutrition is what empowers us to lead rich, fulfilling lives. By understanding and employing the symbiosis of Yoga and Superfoods, we afford ourselves a chance to not just live, but thrive. With the wisdom of the ancients, the bounty of the garden, and the tenacity of the human spirit, achieving optimal health is indeed within our grasp.

Chapter 4. From Mat to Table: Synchronizing Yoga and Nutrition

Practicing yoga cultivates a strong connection with the inner self. To magnify this connection and utilize it to accomplish astonishing feats of wellness and longevity, one must understand the role of nutrition. From the yoga mat to the dining table, entering the realm of healthy living is a delightful adventure teeming with vibrant colors, enticing flavours, and profound wisdom.

4.1. The Yoga Philosophy and Its Correlation to Nutrition

The yoga philosophy extends beyond the mat, permeating every action, thought, and choice we make, including our dietary habits. The ancient philosophy of yoga is deeply rooted in 'Ahimsa' or non-harming. Ahimsa reminds us to consciously choose nourishing foods that cause the least harm to other living beings and the environment.

Simultaneously, yoga emphasizes the concept of 'Sattva' or purity. Sattvic foods, according to yoga philosophy, are pure, clean, and abundant with life force energy. These foods are often plant-based and minimally processed, making them perfect for providing the body with vitality and supporting meditation and yoga practices.

Yoga also directs our attention yoke mind, body, and spirit. In the context of nutrition, this syncs our choices with mindful consumption, balance, moderation, gratitude, and conscious preparation.

4.2. The Science: Digestion, Yoga and Nutrition

It's widely accepted in the scientific community that the gut is the root to overall well-being. Our digestive systems, home to trillions of gut flora, significantly affect our physical health, mood, and cognitive function.

From a purely scientific perspective, yoga exercises significantly enhance digestion. Poses like the 'Ardha Matsyendrasana' (seated twist) and 'Pavanamuktasana' (knees-to-chest pose) can stimulate digestion and help detoxify the body. Coupled with a rich, nutritious diet high in fiber, enzymes, and probiotics, these practices take us many steps closer to vibrant health.

4.3. The Super Duo: Yoga and Superfoods

Regular yoga practices increase the body's demand for nutrients. Superfoods, nutritionally dense and packed with antioxidants, vitamins, and minerals, can dramatically boost health and energy.

Incorporating superfoods into your diet post-yoga nourishes the body. Excellent examples are blueberries, chia seeds, kale, goji berries, raw cacao, and quinoa. These foods provide high-quality nutrients for recovery and rejuvenation, making the body more resilient and helping maintain focus and tranquillity of the mind.

4.4. Synchronizing Yoga and Nutrition: A Practical Guide

Beginning daily routines with yoga primes the body for optimal nutrient absorption. Here is a simple yet effective guide for synchronizing yoga and nutrition:

1. Start the day with a glass of room temperature or slightly warm water. It hydrates the body, jumpstarts metabolism, and aids in flushing out toxins.

2. Practice morning yoga on an empty stomach for maximum efficiency. Light yoga postures can help stimulate your digestive system and kickstart your day.

3. Break your fast with a smoothie packed with superfoods. Try a blend of spinach, chia seeds, almond milk, and a banana.

4. Throughout the day, maintain hydration. Include herbal teas like green tea or peppermint tea which are remarkable for digestion.

5. Have a colorful lunch. Include a variety of vegetables, whole grains, lean protein, and a handful of nuts for optimal energy levels.

6. Avoid eating a heavy meal right before your bedtime yoga practice. If you're hungry, opt for a light snack like some almonds or an apple.

7. Following nighttime yoga, end your day with an infusion of chamomile tea to promote relaxation and sound sleep.

While it seems overwhelming at first, incorporating these practices into daily routines eventually feels natural, and the vibrant results are well worth the effort.

4.5. The Yoga-Superfood Recipes for Vitality and Longevity

Creating dishes filled with superfoods that complement your yoga practice is a delightful gastronomical journey. Here are two simple recipes you can begin with:

4.5.1. Energizing Morning Smoothie

Ingredients:

- 1 handful of spinach or kale
- 1 banana
- 1 tablespoon chia or flax seeds
- 1 tablespoon raw almond butter
- 1 cup of almond milk

Blend all ingredients until smooth. This nutritious concoction provides sustained energy for your morning yoga session and a kickstart to your day.

4.5.2. Healing Turmeric and Ginger Tea

Ingredients:

- 1-inch piece of fresh ginger, finely chopped
- 1-inch piece of fresh turmeric, finely chopped (or 1 teaspoon of turmeric powder)
- 1 teaspoon of honey
- Juice of half a lemon
- 2 cups of water

Boil water with ginger and turmeric for about 10 minutes. Strain and add lemon and honey to taste. It's a healing, rejuvenating delight and a perfect ally for your nighttime yoga session.

Synchronizing yoga with nutrition reaps exponential benefits, leading to a life of vitality, emotional balance, and mental clarity. Each step taken in this journey brings you closer to a wholesome way of living, making peace, joy, and health your constant companions.

Embrace the transformation, and feel yourself bloom into your best self, radiant with health and vitality.

Chapter 5. Kale and Asanas: Superfoods and Yoga Basics

Healthy eating and regular physical activity are key elements of a balanced lifestyle. But when combined with the practice of yoga, superfoods like kale can elevate your health to levels you never thought possible. In this chapter, we zoom in on the fusion of yoga and kale, and how this synergy unlocks profound health benefits and ushers you into the world of optimal well-being.

5.1. Embracing Yoga: An Ancient Practice Rooted in Wellness

Greek philosopher Socrates once said, "An unexamined life is not worth living", and yoga provides just the right tools to help us delve deeper into the self, allowing us to discover our true spirit and awaken our hidden strengths.

The year-old practice of yoga presents a philosophy that goes beyond mere physical postures or asanas. It revolves around the concept of creating and preserving a balance in life — physical, mental, emotional, and spiritual. This system of personal growth helps to develop a sense of self-awareness and fosters inner peace, thus promoting general health and well-being.

5.2. Aspects of Yoga Practice: Asanas and Pranayama

Yoga is traditionally structured around two main components: Asanas and Pranayama.

Asanas, or poses, are designed to improve strength, flexibility, and balance. They're a powerful tool when used properly, but it's essential to select ones that best match your fitness level and personal health goals. Common examples of asanas include Tadasana (Mountain Pose), Trikonasana (Triangle Pose), and Bakasana (Crane Pose).

Pranayama, on the other hand, is the practice of controlling and directing the breath, integral for revitalizing the body and quieting the mind. Some well-known Pranayamas include Anulom Vilom (Alternate Nostril Breathing), Kapalabhati (Skull Shining Breath), and Ujjayi (Ocean Breath).

5.3. Superfood Spotlight: The Power of Kale

Many food choices can play a pivotal role in your overall health, but not all carry the 'superfood' label. Superfoods are nutrient powerhouses with large doses of antioxidants, polyphenols, vitamins, and minerals.

Kale, a part of the cabbage family, is one superfood that towers over the rest. Known for its health-promoting qualities, kale is packed with vitamins A, K, C, and B6, as well as manganese, calcium, copper, potassium, and magnesium. The dense nutrient content of this leafy green can improve skin health, enhance digestion, boost the immune system, and even promote heart health!

5.4. Yoga Meets Kale: Life-changing Synergy

Bringing together the ancient wisdom of yoga and the nutrition-laden composition of kale may seem like an unlikely pairing, but this combination provides a holistic approach that extends far beyond mundane health improvements.

Starting your day with a yoga routine followed by a nutrient-packed kale smoothie, for instance, can keep you energized throughout the day. Adding kale to your diet, along with the tranquility yoga brings, can help reduce stress levels. If you're struggling with insomnia, the calming effect of a yoga practice complemented by a kale-infused dinner can lead to better sleep patterns.

But the journey doesn't end here. The amalgamation of yoga and kale can act as a catalyst for holistic lifestyle changes, steering you towards improved food choices, better stress management, and heightened self-awareness.

5.5. Sequencing with Kale: Combining Yoga and Nutrition

Getting started with integrating the power duo of yoga and kale into your routine doesn't have to be challenging. Here are some easy steps:

1. Begin your day with Surya Namaskar (Sun Salutation), followed by a green smoothie made using kale, bananas, and a hint of lemon.

2. Integrate kale into meals; try swapping out lettuce in your salad with kale, or adding chopped kale to your soup.

3. Practice Pranayama techniques for 10 minutes in the evening; this can enhance digestion, helping your body better assimilate the nutrients from the kale.

4. Prepare a simple kale-based dinner, like a kale and quinoa bowl, and end your evening with restorative asanas like Savasana (Corpse Pose) or Viparita Karani (Legs-Up-The-Wall).

5.6. Taking the Plunge: The Yoga-Kale Lifestyle

Embracing this new way of life—a harmonious blend of asanas, pranayama, and kale—can be a significant game-changer in your journey towards optimal health. As yoga guru B.K.S. Iyengar said, "Health is a state of complete harmony of the body, mind, and spirit." So, it's time to dive in. Let this fusion of yoga and super-nourishment from kale be your stepping-stone towards achieving this harmony. Let the ultimate symbiosis of mind, body, and nutrition begin!

Just remember, consistency is crucial in this journey as it helps to sustain the transformations you've achieved, ensuring that your journey towards wellbeing is not just a fleeting episode, but a lifelong narrative of health and contentment.

Chapter 6. Deep Dive into Yoga: Demystifying Styles and Poses for Health

Yoga, an ancient practice steeped in over 5,000 years of history, serves as a holistic tool for achieving optimal health. It encompasses elaborate sequences of physical poses, meditation, breath work, and ethical standards, all of which imbue the practitioner with an array of benefits, ranging from physical strength and flexibility to mental tranquility and spiritual enlightenment.

6.1. Understanding the Power of Yoga

Our physical bodies are inextricably interconnected with our mental, emotional, and spiritual selves, in a continuous cycle of mutual effect. Yoga seeks to harmonize and balance these aspects, inducing a state of wholeness. It is also seen as a bridge between the mind and body – a pathway to unite our outer, material existence with our inner, spiritual self.

The physical poses or asanas, mindful breathing or pranayama, and meditation practices in yoga can enhance bodily fitness, relieve stress, improve mood, and boost cognitive function. Regular yoga practice can also alleviate chronic health issues like insomnia, depression, low back pain, and can even aid in weight loss.

6.2. Yoga Styles: A Comparative Analysis

Numerous yoga styles exist, each with unique characteristics catering to a diverse range of preferences. Some of the well-known styles are:

- **Hatha:** Regarded as a vital class for beginners, Hatha Yoga includes basic postures and focuses primarily on breath control and meditation. This approach is often slower-paced, paving the way for an enriched understanding of each pose.

- **Vinyasa:** Often referred to as 'flow yoga', Vinyasa includes a dynamic series of poses in which each movement corresponds to a breath. This form focuses on developing strength and flexibility and is more vigorous compared to Hatha Yoga.

- **Ashtanga:** This style is a fast-paced intensive method characterized by six strictly fixed series of poses executed in sequential order. Ashtanga enhances endurance, flexibility, and strength, making it suitable for advanced practitioners.

- **Yin:** Yin Yoga targets our deep connective tissues, such as the fascia, ligaments, joints, and bones. It's slower and more meditative, providing you the space to turn inward and tune into both your mind and the physical sensations of your body.

- **Restorative:** A style designed to relax and restore the body. It utilizes props to allow you to stay in poses for a longer duration, fostering deep relaxation and healing.

6.3. The Impact of Selected Yoga Poses

Let's delve into the benefits of some common yoga poses and how to incorporate them in your daily routine:

- **Mountain Pose (Tadasana):** The foundation for all other poses, Mountain Pose improves posture, balance and calm focus. Simply stand tall, press your weight evenly across both feet, tuck your tailbone in and roll your shoulders back.

- **Downward-Facing Dog (Adho Mukha Svanasana):** This

effective full-body stretch improves flexibility in the hamstrings and calves, strengthens the shoulders, and reduces stress. Start on your hands and knees, and then lift your knees off the floor, straightening your legs as you push your heels towards the floor.

- **Warrior II (Virabhadrasana II):** A powerful standing pose that tones the legs and core while expanding the chest and shoulders. Stand tall, step one foot back and angle it outward, then bend the front knee and stretch your arms out to the sides.

- **Tree Pose (Vrksasana):** Excellent for improving balance, strengthening the core and legs, and promoting a sense of calm. Stand tall, shift your weight onto one leg, then place the other foot on to the inner thigh or calf of the standing leg. Extend your arms overhead.

Regular practice of these poses could help enhance your physical and mental well-being, becoming the cornerstone to a richer, more vibrant life.

6.4. Integrating Yoga into Your Daily Life

Incorporating yoga into your daily routine does not need to be daunting. Start simple, with just a few minutes per day, and gradually increase the duration as you build strength and flexibility. Here are a few implementation tips:

1. Start with a quiet, distraction-free space.

2. Set regular practice times that accommodate your schedule.

3. Use quality yoga equipment, like a mat and comfortable clothing.

4. Listen to your body and adjust poses to fit your abilities.

5. Consider joining a yoga class or finding a mentor for guidance.

Being patient and consistent is key. Keeping an open mind and heart to the teachings of yoga can influence not only physical health but also mental state, emotional well-being, and an enriched spiritual life.

Unleash the power of the ultimate synergy of yoga and superfoods, as you journey on your path to peak health and wellness. Cultivate a mindful connection between your bodily sensations, emotions, and thoughts. Let the legacy of yogic wisdom lead your transformation towards radiant health and unparalleled longevity.

Chapter 7. Superfoods Unleashed: Navigating Nutritional Powerhouses

We take a deep-dive into the world of superfoods, exploring their benefits, how to choose them, and how to integrate them into your lifestyle. A word of advice before you embark on this journey: Do not sprint but rather take measured strides. The goal is to integrate these nutritionally dense heroes into your meals slowly but consistently.

7.1. Knowing Your Superfoods

Superfoods are nutrient powerhouses that pack large doses of antioxidants, polyphenols, vitamins, and minerals. Regular consumption of these foods could improve your lifespan, reduce your risk of chronic diseases, and help you maintain a healthy weight.

Critical to discern is that no single food, not even a superfood, can offer all the nutrition, health benefits, and energy we need to nourish our bodies. A balanced diet incorporating a variety of superfoods will help you gain the maximum health benefits.

Let's explore some of these superstars of the food world!

7.2. A Kaleidoscope of Superfoods

Blueberries: The antioxidant-rich berries are believed to delay brain aging and improve memory.

Broccoli: This cruciferous vegetable is high in fibre and contains multiple nutrients with potent anti-cancer properties.

Chia Seeds: Packed with a huge amount of nutrients and very few calories, these tiny seeds are loaded with antioxidants, high-quality protein, and omega-3 fatty acids.

Goji Berries: These berries are excellent sources of Vitamin C and antioxidants.

Quinoa: This grain is high in protein and is one of the few plant foods that contain all nine essential amino acids.

Sweet Potatoes: They offer a healthy dose of fiber, as well as an array of vitamins and minerals, such as iron, calcium, selenium, and they are a good source of most of our B vitamins and vitamin C.

7.3. Harmonizing Them Into Your Meals

Begin by adding one superfood to your diet at a time. Allow your body to adjust before adding another. Discover which superfoods you relish, and which you'd rather avoid.

7.4. Experimenting With Recipes

Having superfoods doesn't mean you are restricted to eating them raw or steamed. For example, you could toss blueberries or goji berries in your salad for an antioxidant-rich meal. Experiment to make things exciting!

7.5. Superfood Smoothies

Another fantastic way of incorporating superfoods into your meals is through smoothies. A spinach, blueberry, banana, and almond milk smoothie can become a regular breakfast item.

7.6. Storing Superfoods

Storing superfoods correctly will ensure they maintain their nutrient content. Store grains and seeds in air-tight containers. Refrigerate fruits and vegetables promptly.

7.7. Superfood Supplements

You can also consider superfood supplements. However, remember that these should never replace meals. Their purpose is to supplement a healthy diet, not substitute it.

As you embrace superfoods, remember that balanced nutrition is key. Combining these nutrition powerhouses with a regular exercise regimen, and loads of hydration, you're one step ahead on your wellness journey.

But, there's more! With our next chapter, we'll introduce you to the magic of yoga and how it creates an exceptional duo with superfoods for an overall harmonious lifestyle. So, Stay tuned!

This journey of embracing superfoods might seem overwhelming initially, but remember, the road to a healthy lifestyle is about taking small, consistent steps. Begin today, one superfood at a time.

Chapter 8. Recipe for Radiance: Superfood Recipes for Yogis

The yogic journey is marked by a commitment to nurturing one's body, mind, and spirit. One key avenue for this nurturing is through eating, and what is more nourishing than superfoods? Superfoods, being nutrient-dense foods, can provide your body with the vitamins, minerals, and antioxidants it needs to function at its best. While practicing yoga helps improve flexibility, strength, and mental well-being, pairing it with a diet abundant in superfoods can boost your health and vitality even further.

8.1. Superfoods: Defining the Powerhouses

Superfoods are foods—mostly plant-based but also some fish and dairy—known for being nutrient powerhouses. They pack large doses of antioxidants, polyphenols, vitamins, and minerals. And when incorporated into your diet, can improve energy, aid in disease prevention and promote a healthier lifestyle.

Let's explore some of these superfoods and how they can be a part of your yogic diet.

8.2. Berries

Berries are rich in antioxidants and vitamin C, both of which can help reduce inflammation, boost immunity, and keep your skin healthy. You can enjoy them fresh in the summer and frozen during the other seasons.

Example Recipe: Berry Boost Smoothie

Ingredients

* 1 cup of mixed berries (like blueberries,
strawberries, and raspberries)
* 1 cup of unsweetened almond milk
* 1 tablespoon of chia seeds
* A handful of spinach or kale
* Ice cubes

Method

1. Add all the ingredients to a blender.
2. Blend until smooth.
3. Serve immediately.

8.3. Leafy Greens

Leafy greens such as kale, spinach, and Swiss chard are full of
essential vitamins and minerals which help to improve your energy
levels.

Example Recipe: Leafy Green Delight Salad

Ingredients

* 2 cups of mixed greens (spinach, kale, and arugula)
* 1/2 cup of cherry tomatoes, halved
* 1/2 avocado, sliced
* 1/4 cup of walnuts
* 1 tablespoon of olive oil
* 1 tablespoon of balsamic vinegar
* Salt and pepper to taste

Method

1. Combine the greens, cherry tomatoes, avocado, and
walnuts in a large bowl.
2. In a small bowl, whisk together the olive oil,
balsamic vinegar, salt, and pepper.
3. Drizzle the dressing over the salad and toss to
combine.

8.4. Super Seeds

Seeds, like chia, flax, and hemp, are high in fiber and omega-3 fatty
acids, which may support heart health and curb your appetite.

Example Recipe: Seed-Powered Overnight Oats

Ingredients

* 1/2 cup of rolled oats
* 1 cup of almond milk
* 1 tablespoon of chia seeds
* 1 tablespoon of flax seeds
* 1/2 banana, sliced
* A handful of chopped nuts (like almond, walnuts)
* A drizzle of honey or maple syrup

Method

1. In a jar, combine the oats, almond milk, chia seeds,
and flax seeds.
2. Stir until mixed and refrigerate overnight.
3. In the morning, top with sliced banana, chopped nuts,
and a drizzle of your chosen sweetener.

Embrace these recipes as part of your yogic journey to wellness and deeper connection with your body. The satisfying flavors and nutrient-dense ingredients can empower you and assist towards lasting health and well-being. Remember, balance is key. Practice regular yoga and mindfully nourish your body. And soon, you'll be radiating with vibrant health – from within and without.

Chapter 9. A Day in the Life: Daily Routines for Harmonious Living

A mindful and intentional approach to your daily routine is a powerful guide to harmonious living. By integrating nutritious superfoods and yoga practices into your day, you can experience immense benefits from enhanced energy levels to superior well-being.

9.1. Morning

Embarking on your day with a balanced combination of mind, body, and nutrition activities can set the pace for a day filled with harmonious living.

Wake up early when it's quieter and nature sounds begin to fill the air for a morning yoga session. Rineties like the Sun Salutation sequence are perfect for this time, invigorating your energy and waking up your muscles. This multistep sequence helps to develop the strength and flexibility of the entire body, all while synchronizing your movements with your breath.

On your breakfast plate, consider superfoods packed with nutrients to fuel your workout and day. A green smoothie is an excellent candidate. Blend the power duo of spinach - rich in iron, calcium, and vitamins K, A, and C - and kale, a vitamin powerhouse, with a banana for creaminess, chia seeds for fiber and omega-3, and fresh apple juice. This vibrant glassful is a nutrient bomb that's both delicious and energy-boosting.

9.2. Mid-Morning

Nourish your mid-morning hours with a routine that aligns your mind, body, and food.

Taking breaks to perform yoga, even for just five minutes to stretch, can help to refresh both your mind and body. Chair Yoga, for instance, can help you relieve stress without leaving your workstation. This is an adaptation of traditional yoga poses that can be done while seated in a chair.

Converge your mid-morning snack with superfood. Almonds, walnuts or brazil nuts are go-to choices. Each is dense in vitamins and minerals, fiber and protein, and they promote heart health.

9.3. Afternoon

Your afternoon routine is an excellent opportunity to recharge your body and feed your soul with the right nutrition.

Post meal yoga can aid your digestion. Yoga poses like Seated Forward Bend, Knees-to-Chest pose, or Supine Twist are gentle and work well.

For lunch, consider a quinoa salad loaded with veggies like cucumber and bell peppers, avocado cubes, and a punch of protein with sprouted legumes or grilled tofu, with a dressing of olive oil, lemon juice, and peppery arugula. Quinoa, tofu, and avocado are superfoods celebrated for their significant health benefits.

9.4. Evening

As the day edges towards its end, yoga and soup are ideal for a grounding and peaceful evening.

Restorative yoga poses like the Child's Pose or Legs-up-the-Wall pose are great options. Such poses encourage slower movements and deep, relaxed breathing, getting you ready for a tranquil night.

For dinner, nourishing soups with superfoods like broccoli, carrots, sweet potatoes, chickpeas, and with a topping of protein-rich amaranth seeds can offer a warm, comforting end to the day.

9.5. Night

A pre-bed ritual incorporates calming yoga and nutrient-rich superfood.

Yoga before bedtime can help ease your body and mind into a state of peace after a long day. Try a couple of soothing poses such as the Corpse Pose or Reclined Butterfly pose.

Consider a golden milk - a blend of almond milk, turmeric, a pinch of black pepper and a dollop of honey as a superfood nightcap. It is promising for its anti-inflammatory and antioxidant properties and its aid in promoting weighted sleep.

Incorporate this comprehensive day plan to your daily life, imbibe the powerful effects of yoga and superfood, and blossom into a life of harmonious living.

Chapter 10. Tips and Tricks for a Balanced Yogic Diet

Beyond simply promoting physical fitness, yoga and mindful eating go hand in hand in fostering an overall sense of health, vitality, and inner tranquility. The ancient principles of a balanced yogic diet encourage a holistic immersion into wellbeing that stretches beyond the yoga mat. By mindfully incorporating specific superfoods into our diet, we can optimize the transformative benefits of our yoga practice, augment our energy levels, bolster our immune system, and elevate our conscious connection with our bodies.

10.1. Understanding the Yogic Diet

Yoga, a practiced discipline from ancient India, fosters harmonious integration of body, mind, and spirit. A cornerstone of this integrative philosophy includes the concept of 'Ahimsa' or non-violence, interpreted not only as behavior towards others but also towards oneself. Therefore, a yogic diet encourages gentle, nurturing, health-affirming sustenance.

In Ayurveda, an ancient medical science that yoga embraces, everything we eat is converted into energy or 'prana'—life force. Food possessing high 'prana' principles include fresh, organic fruits, vegetables, grains, legumes, nuts, seeds, and superfoods—nutritionally dense foods brimming with vitamins, minerals, antioxidants, and other health-enhancing compounds.

Balancing the 'Gunas' or qualities, 'Sattva' (purity), 'Rajas' (activity, passion), and 'Tamas' (darkness, inertia) in food is also crucial. A Sattvic diet comprising whole, freshly prepared foods brings clarity, understanding, and spiritual growth, aiding yoga practitioners to settle into calming, deep, meditative states.

10.2. Incorporating Superfoods into a Yogic Diet

Embedding superfoods into a yogic diet amps up the nutritional value, optimizes yoga benefits, and promotes a healthy body. Here's the roster of select superfoods, along with their health benefits:

1. **Goji Berries:** Long revered in China, these tiny powerhouses with bright hues are packed rich with antioxidants and Vitamin C. They also support the immune system and enhance the skin's youthful glow.

2. **Chia Seeds:** These tiny seeds are rich in Omega-3 fatty acids, protein, fiber, calcium, and antioxidants. Known for their energy-boosting properties, they may enhance endurance, helping yoga practitioners hold asanas longer.

3. **Quinoa:** This whole grain superfood is a complete protein rich in various vitamins, minerals, and fibers. It aids digestion and provides sustained energy for prolonged yogic practices.

4. **Kale:** A nutrient-dense leafy green packed with vitamins A, K, C, B6, and various minerals. It supports bone health, promotes healthy skin, and assists in detoxification.

5. **Blueberries:** Rich in antioxidants, fiber, and Vitamin C, these sweet berries promote a healthy heart, support brain health, maintain skin health, and aid weight management.

10.3. Pre and Post Yoga Meals

Incorporating the right foods at the right time can significantly fuel your yoga practice and recovery, helping you reap maximum health benefits.

Pre-Yoga Nutrition: Eating a light, easily digestible meal at least two hours before your yoga session is recommended. This could be a smoothie made with bananas, blueberries, spinach, and a spoon of chia seeds, or a slice of whole-grain toast with almond butter.

Post-Yoga Nutrition: Rehydrate and replenish lost nutrients post-yoga with a substantial, balanced meal. A bowl of cooked quinoa, sautéed kale, roasted sweet potatoes, topped with goji berries makes an excellent recovery meal.

10.4. Simple Recipes for a Yogic Diet

Tasty, easy-to-make recipes using superfoods further fortify a yogic diet while catering to your taste buds.

Chia Seed Pudding: Soak 3 tablespoons of chia seeds in a cup of almond milk overnight. In the morning, stir in your favorite fruits, nuts, or seeds.

Quinoa Salad: Cook quinoa as per instructions and let it cool. Mix in cherry tomatoes, cucumber, feta cheese, and fresh herbs. Drizzle with olive oil, lemon juice, salt, and pepper. Toss and serve.

Goji Berry Tea: Soak a handful of goji berries in hot water for around 10 minutes, until they become plump. Enjoy the tea as it is or mixed with a bit of honey.

10.5. Mindful Eating: A Yogic Approach Beyond the Plate

The practice of yoga impresses upon the harmony between mind, body, and spirit, which can be extended to our eating habits. Mindful eating—eating with attention, savoring every morsel, chewing thoroughly, expressing gratitude for the food, and acknowledging the nourishment it provides—promotes optimum digestion, satiety, and opens the door to healthier food choices and eating behaviors. This invaluable practice makes us creators of our health and wellbeing, adding another level of depth to a yogic lifestyle.

In conclusion, a balanced yogic diet incorporating superfoods acts like a force multiplier in respect of the overall health benefits accrued from practicing yoga. Healthy dietary practices coupled with yoga ensure a fit body, a tranquil mind, and a nourished soul—an unparalleled symbiotic relationship promoting radiant vitality and longevity. Investing in this lifestyle is the most rewarding step towards optimal health, ensuring the journey to peak wellness is as pleasurable as the destination itself.

Chapter 11. Journey Continues: Maintaining Your New Lifestyle

Having discovered the quest for a well-rounded approach to health that comprehends both yoga and superfoods, it's imperative to acknowledge the need for maintaining this newly adopted lifestyle. It might seem like a daunting task initially, but the investment of effort and consistency is soon exceeded by the iridescent benefits.

11.1. Embracing the Path of Continual Learning

As you plunge deeper into your journey with yoga and superfoods, remember that the journey itself is an education. Stickiness is seasoned by a persistent learner's mindset. Even as you grow more adept with yoga poses or surprise yourself with a creative superfood recipe, keep an open mind to learning new techniques, undiscovered foods, and unique health benefits. Lifestyle changes require perseverance, openness and knowledge. Books, scholarly articles, dieticians, and skilled yoga instructors are excellent resources to tap into. Remember, the power couple – yoga and superfoods, is an expansive universe.

11.2. Building a Personalized Life Schedule

One of the most efficient ways to ensure the maintenance of your new lifestyle is to establish a structure that accommodates it. Carve out a regular time slot for your yoga practice. As for the assimilation of superfoods, craft a weekly meal plan. Try to include at least one superfood every day initially, and slowly work your way up. Introduce substitutes instead of complete overhauls. For example, snack on blueberries instead of chips, or begin your day with quinoa breakfast bowls.

11.3. Making Incremental Changes

Change doesn't emerge all at once, nor is it expected from you. It's all about taking small steps and settling them into your daily routine. This approach is far more realistic and less overwhelming. Only when you feel ready do you move onto the next change. Be patient with yourself and take time to appreciate the progress you make, no matter how small it seems.

11.4. Regular Practice of Yoga

Yoga is more than just physical exercise; it's a holistic experience. To deeply embed this discipline into your life, you need to regularly commit to it. Not only should you practice the poses but it's essential to meditate and engage in breathing exercises. As these practices are not strenuous, they can be enjoyed daily. Consistency is the key. Consider joining a yoga community for encouragement and motivation.

11.5. Experimenting with Superfoods

To foster a lasting relationship with superfoods, incorporate variety. A single superfood isn't the narrative here. Explore indigenous vegetables, exotic fruits, and protein-rich grains. Experiment with diverse recipes that make these healthy foods delicious. You can start baking with almond flour, or make a spirulina smoothie. Your culinary adventure with superfoods will keep your palate tingling and your body flourishing.

11.6. Staying Motivated

The maintenance of your lifestyle is tethered by motivation. Remember why you began this journey and what accomplishments you'd like to reap. Celebrate milestones, no matter how small. Also, occasional yoga retreats or cooking workshops can keep the enthusiasm lively.

11.7. Prep for Bumps

On the road to a lifestyle change, there will be challenges. Occasional failures should not deter you from your journey. Accept these, learn from them, and keep moving forward.

11.8. The Power of Accountability

Having a yoga partner or cooking buddy can make this journey more exciting. When you commit to someone, the chances of sticking with your new lifestyle grow higher. Also, social media can serve as an excellent platform for accountability, inspiration, and community building.

11.9. Changing from the Inside

As you progress, be ready to feel the transformation from within. Positive lifestyle changes often come with higher energy levels, improved sleep, greater self-confidence, and overall better health.

In conclusion, envisaging a lifestyle change is step one to a healthier life. Implementing it is step two, and maintaining is the cherry on top! It's an iterative process, much like life itself. Enjoy the journey as you continue to navigate these exciting realms of yoga and superfoods.